The Alkaline Diet for Hair Growth

A comprehensive guide for using alkaline recipes to combat hair loss, balding, dandruff, and infections of the scalp.

Dr. Amalie Kleist

Table of Contents

DISCLAIMER

This content is not meant to offer medical advice or replace advice or treatment from a personal physician. It is recommended that you get advice from your doctors or trained health specialists for any specific health inquiries you may have. Readers or followers of this instructional resource are responsible for any potential health effects.

Introduction

Enter a world where the possibilities for your hair are endless! Presenting "The Alkaline Diet for Hair Growth," an innovative piece of creativity by the renowned Dr. Amalie Kleist that reveals the keys to unleashing your hair's luminosity like never before.

In a society that frequently refers to hair as our crowning glory, Dr. Kleist's knowledge is evident as she explores the transformative impact of the alkaline diet. Through a thorough investigation and a strong interest in holistic health, she reveals a revolutionary approach to hair care that goes beyond traditional practices. Imagine having hair that radiates vigor, tenacity, and irresistible charm every morning as you wake up.

The book by Dr. Kleist is more than simply a how-to manual; it's a ray of hope for everyone hoping to bring their hair journey back to life. Through the lens of alkalinity, she sheds light on the complex relationship between diet and hair health, showing how a pH balance can serve as the foundation for your hair's revival.

This book isn't like other diet books. A manifesto of empowerment, "The Alkaline Diet for Hair Growth," provides readers with a road map for taking back control of their hair's future. Bid farewell to the annoyance of boring locks and welcome to a renewed sense of inner confidence. Utilizing an abundance of scientific knowledge and years of expertise, Dr. Kleist demystifies hair care and offers doable solutions that everyone can include in their daily practice. This book is filled with practical advice that will revitalize your hair, ranging from little food modifications to focused lifestyle improvements. But it's about more than simply aesthetics—it's about taking back your identity. You'll go on a life-changing adventure that goes beyond outward beauty with Dr. Kleist as your guide, encouraging a closer bond between mind, body, and soul. Are you prepared to accept the robust, lustrous hair you've always deserved? Go on an unmatched journey of self-discovery, empowerment, and transformation with Dr. Amalie Kleist.

This is where your hair's next chapter begins!

Chapter One

Human hair basics

Hair appears simpler than it actually is. You may feel it at the root when it moves or is pulled. It keeps dust and other particles out of your eyes and ears, while also shielding your skin. Your hairdo can serve as a means of self-expression. When your hair becomes damaged, it has the ability to regenerate itself without leaving any permanent marks. Hair covers the human body nearly entirely.

Human hair is a complex biological characteristic that serves multiple purposes and has cultural importance in many countries. Here are a few basic principles for human hair:

A morphological description of hair

The morphological description of human hair entails an examination of its physical attributes and internal composition. Here is a comprehensive analysis:

LENGTH: The length of human hair can range from several feet to a few millimeters, with a wide variation among individuals.

COLOR: The concentration and type of melanin pigments found in the cortex layer of the hair shaft determine its color. Melanin can exist in two forms: eumelanin, which results in the production of black or brown colors, and pheomelanin, which leads to the production of yellow or red colors. The combination of these pigments results in a diverse spectrum of hair hues, spanning from fair-haired to dark-haired, with a multitude of intermediate tints.

TEXTURE: Texture pertains to the thickness or diameter of individual hair filaments. We can categorize it as fine, medium, or coarse. Texture encompasses the arrangement of waves or curls in the hair, which can range from straight to wavy, curly, or kinky.

SHAPE: You can find different hair shafts with varying cross-sectional shapes. The shape of the object can vary between round, oval, or irregular. The shape of the hair has an impact on its visual characteristics and behavior, including its curl pattern and vulnerability to harm.

CUTICLE: The cuticle is the hair shaft's outermost layer. A series of scales that overlap and lie flat shield the hair, protecting the underlying layers. The state of the cuticle directly impacts the hair's luster, sleekness, and ability to withstand harm.

CORTEX: The cortex is the middle layer of the hair shaft. It is made up of long cells that are filled with keratin proteins and pigment granules. It imparts the hair with durability, flexibility, and pigmentation.

MEDULLA: In human hair, the medulla, the innermost layer of the hair shaft, is not always present. If it is present, it consists of loosely packed cells and air voids. The precise role of this substance in human hair remains unclear, and its size and visibility can differ across individuals.

ROOT AND SHAFT: The hair root is the part of the hair that lies beneath the skin's surface within the hair follicle. The hair shaft, which extends above the surface of the epidermis, is visible to the naked eye.

DENSITY: Hair density is the measure of the number of individual hair strands per square inch of the scalp. The variations in people can have an impact on their overall volume and thickness of hair.

The Hair's Structure

A single strand of hair may appear simple, but it is one of the body's most complex systems. Hair consists of two distinct components. The hair follicle is located below the skin, while the hair shaft is visible above the skin.

HAIR FOLLICLE

The hair follicle serves as the starting point for hair development and its retention in place. The structure in question is a stocking-like formation that originates in the epidermis, which is the outermost layer of the skin. It extends to the dermis, which is the second layer of your skin.

The papilla, located at the base of the follicle, consists of small blood vessels known as capillaries. These substances provide essential nutrients to the hair follicle, promoting its continuous growth. The follicle also houses the germinal matrix, which is responsible for the production of new hairs.

The bulb is a spherical structure located within the skin, specifically at the hair's base, which encloses the papilla and germinal matrix. The organism possesses many types of stem cells that differentiate into specialized cells and have the ability to self-renew over an extended period of time.

The follicle is encased by both an inner and outer sheath, which serve to shield and shape the developing hair. The inner sheath goes along with the hair and ends just before the oil gland, also known as the sebaceous gland, opens. The outer covering extends fully to the gland.

The sebaceous gland secretes sebum, often known as oil, which serves as the body's innate conditioner. Puberty leads to an increased production of sebum, resulting in the prevalence of acne during adolescence. The production of sebum reduces as one ages, resulting in the skin becoming dry.

The arrector pili muscle, a small cluster of muscle fibers, is connected to the outer layer. Contraction of the muscle leads to the phenomenon of hair standing up, commonly referred to as goose bumps.

HAIR SHAFT

The term "hair shaft" refers to the visible portion of hair. When hair grows beyond the skin's surface, the cells no longer function. The structure consists of three layers composed of keratin, a protein that undergoes hardening. The layers are as follows:

- **The Inner Layer:** This is known as the medulla. The medulla's presence varies depending on the hair type.

- **The Middle Layer:** This is known as the cortex, it comprises the majority of the hair shaft.

Pigmenting cells, located in the medulla and cortex, are responsible for hair coloration.

- **The Outer Layer:** This is the cuticle, and it is made up of tightly packed scales that overlap in a way that looks like roof shingles. Several hair conditioning solutions are designed to cleanse the cuticle by enhancing its smoothness and structure.

The Hair Growth Cycle

The hair on your scalp grows at a rate of less than 0.5 millimeters every day. Individual hairs are always growing in one of three stages: anagen, catagen, or telogen.

STAGE 1: ANAGEN PHASE (GROWTH STAGE)

The anagen phase is the time when hair grows. This period lasts for several years for most hair types. The old hair that has finished growing out of the follicle is pushed out by new hair. For leg and arm hair, eyebrows, and eyelashes, the anagen phase lasts only 30 to 45 days. That's why those hairs are usually shorter than the ones on your head.

- *Duration:* Depending on a number of variables like age, general health, and heredity, this phase may extend for two, six, or even more years.

- *Activity:* Throughout the anagen phase, the hair follicles are actively producing hair. Hair shaft elongation occurs when the hair bulb's cells divide quickly and push older cells upward.

- *Growth Rate:* During the anagen phase, hair grows on average about half an inch (1.25 cm) every month.

- *Hair Percentage:* At any given time, 85–90% of the hair on the scalp is in the anagen phase.

STAGE 2: CATAGEN PHASE (TRANSITIONAL

STAGE)

The catagen phase is a transitional stage that lasts a few weeks and affects 2% of all scalp hairs at any given moment. During this slower growth period, the outer root sheath shrinks and affixes to the hair root. This turns into club hair, which is non-growing hair.

- *Duration:* The catagen phase lasts about two to three weeks.

- *Activity:* This stage is the change from the anagen, or active growth phase, to the telogen, or resting phase. Hair shafts separate from the blood supply, and hair follicles atrophy.

- *Growth Rate:* During the catagen phase, hair growth dramatically slows down.

- *Hair Percentage:* At any given time, only 1-3 percent of the hair on the scalp is in the catagen phase.

STAGE 3: TELOGEN PHASE (RESTING STAGE)

The resting period, known as the telogen phase, lasts for roughly three months. It makes up between 10% and 15% of total hair. The hair follicle is dormant, and the club hair is fully developed during this stage. As the hair pulls out, a white, dry substance is visible at its root.

- *Duration:* The telogen phase lasts for three to four months.

- *Activity:* No new hair growth happens during this phase; instead, the hair follicles are in a resting condition. The old hair remains in the follicle despite its loose attachment to the root.

- *Shedding:* As the telogen phase comes to an end, the old hair sheds, and a new hair development cycle is initiated by the new hair growing underneath it.

- *Hair Percentage:* At any given time, 10–15% of

the hair on the scalp is in the telogen phase.

Hair follicles normally re-enter the anagen phase and begin a fresh round of hair growth after the telogen period, repeating the cycle. It is significant to remember that the growth cycles of individual hair follicles are not completely coordinated. Because of this, different hairs on the scalp are always in different stages of the hair growth cycle, which guarantees that hair is constantly growing. Furthermore, each phase of the hair growth cycle has a different duration and advancement depending on a number of factors, including stress, nutrition, hormones, and heredity.

Chapter Two

Hormonal actions in effective hair growth

Hormones are essential for controlling hair growth and have a significant impact on the hair growth cycle, as well as the thickness, distribution, and patterns of hair. Several crucial hormones have a role in promoting hair development, including:

> **Testosterone and dihydrotestosterone (DHT):**

Testosterone is an androgen hormone principally synthesized in the testes of males and, to a lesser extent, in the ovaries of females. Testosterone promotes the development of facial and body hair throughout adolescence in both males and females.

The enzyme 5-alpha-reductase converts testosterone into

dihydrotestosterone (DHT). Dihydrotestosterone (DHT) is a highly potent androgen that plays a key role in controlling hair development in parts of the body that are sensitive to androgens, such as the scalp. In individuals with a hereditary predisposition to androgenetic alopecia (male-pattern baldness or female-pattern hair loss), dihydrotestosterone (DHT) can attach to hair follicles on the scalp, causing the follicles to shrink and resulting in gradual hair thinning and eventual hair loss.

➢ Estrogens:

The ovaries predominantly synthesize estrogens, the main female sex hormones. They also have significant functions in males, although in lesser amounts. Estrogens exert a beneficial influence on hair growth by extending the anagen phase of the hair growth cycle and enhancing the thickness of hair shafts. During pregnancy, elevated levels of estrogen frequently lead to a temporary increase in hair thickness and a decrease in hair shedding.

Following childbirth, there is a decrease in estrogen levels, which triggers a phase of hair loss called telogen effluvium.

> **Progesterone:**

Progesterone is a female sex hormone that has a role in controlling the menstrual cycle and pregnancy. Although the precise impact of progesterone on hair development is not as well understood as that of estrogen, variations in progesterone levels can indirectly influence hair growth by interacting with other hormones, including estrogen and androgens.

> **Thyroid hormones:**

Thyroid hormones, such as thyroxine (T4) and triiodothyronine (T3), have a vital function in controlling metabolism and energy generation in the body. Thyroid problems, such as hypothyroidism (a condition where the thyroid gland is not producing enough hormones) and hyperthyroidism (a condition where the thyroid gland is producing too many hormones), can interfere with the normal cycle of hair development, resulting in hair loss or thinning. Hair that is fragile, lacking in moisture, and experiencing hair loss specifically correlates with hypothyroidism.

> **Insulin-Like Growth Factor-1 (IGF-1):**

Growth hormone stimulates the liver to synthesize IGF-1.IGF-1 plays a role in the growth and multiplication of cells, including hair follicle cells, during the anagen phase of the hair growth cycle. Inadequate amounts of IGF-1 can result in compromised hair growth.

Optimal hormone management is crucial for sustaining healthy hair growth. Hormonal imbalances or disruptions can interfere with the normal hair development cycle, resulting in a variety of hair problems, including androgenetic alopecia, telogen effluvium, and hormonal hair loss. The individual who is interacting with the system.

The reasons for human hair loss

Numerous factors, including hormone imbalances, genetics, illnesses, drugs, and lifestyle choices, can cause alopecia, the medical term for hair loss. The following are some common causes of human hair loss:

ANDROGENETIC ALOPECIA (MALE AND FEMALE PATTERN BALDNESS)

Genetic predisposition is the main cause of androgenetic alopecia. This disorder usually manifests as widespread hair thinning over the crown area in women, whereas it usually manifests in men as a receding hairline and thinning at the crown.

ANAGEN EFFLUVIUM

Anagen effluvium causes hair loss very quickly. Chemotherapy or radiation treatment are typically to blame for this. After treatment is complete, hair typically grows back.

TELOGEN EFFLUVIUM

Profuse hair shedding characterizes telogen effluvium, a temporary type of hair loss. Many things, including giving birth, major surgery, serious sickness, a lot of stress, or considerable weight loss, might cause it. Telogen effluvium disrupts the regular cycle of hair growth, causing hair follicles to transition from the anagen (growing) phase to the telogen (resting) phase and then shed.

TINEA CAPITIS

A fungal infection that can affect the scalp and hair shaft is known as tinea capitis, sometimes referred to as ringworm of the scalp. It results in tiny, scaly, itchy patches of baldness. If treatment is delayed, the patch or patches will eventually get bigger and fill with pus. These patches, also known as kerions, have the potential to leave scars. Other signs and symptoms include soreness in the scalp, brittle hair that breaks easily, and scaly, reddish-gray areas of skin. It is curable with antifungal medication.

TRACTION ALOPECIA

Excessive strain and tension on the hair, typically caused by wearing it in tight fashions like braids, ponytails, or buns, causes traction alopecia.

ALOPECIA AREATA

Alopecia areata is an autoimmune disorder that can be recognized by the presence of bald patches on the scalp or body. The autoimmune response results in the destruction of hair follicles, causing alopecia. Hereditary factors, stress, or environmental stimuli can trigger it at any stage of life.

MEDICAL CONDITIONS AND TREATMENTS

Certain medical conditions and treatments can cause hair loss as a side effect. Some examples of conditions that might cause hair loss are thyroid problems (namely hypothyroidism and hyperthyroidism), lupus, scalp infections (such as ringworm), trichotillomania (a disorder characterized by compulsive hair pulling), and chemotherapy.

HORMONAL CHANGES

Hormonal fluctuations from pregnancy, childbirth, menopause, or hormonal disorders can cause hair loss. Androgens, specifically dihydrotestosterone (DHT), can cause hair loss in those who are genetically prone to it by shrinking hair follicles, as observed in androgenetic alopecia.

NUTRITIONAL DEFICIENCIES

This includes insufficient consumption of essential minerals such as iron, zinc, vitamin D, and protein, which can be a contributing factor to hair loss. Insufficient intake of essential nutrients can interrupt the natural process of hair growth, resulting in fragile, breakage-prone hair or excessive shedding.

MEDICATIONS

Some treatments, including chemotherapy drugs, beta-blockers, retinoids, anticoagulants, and certain antidepressants, can lead to hair loss as a side effect. The occurrence of hair loss can vary in duration, either temporary or permanent, depending on the specific medication used and the individual's unique reaction.

STRESS

Stress, whether due to physical or mental factors, can induce hair loss by altering the regular hair growth cycle. Stress-induced hair loss may manifest as telogen effluvium or worsen pre-existing hair loss disorders.

Gaining insight into the root cause of hair loss is essential for proper management and treatment. Seeking guidance from a healthcare specialist, such as a dermatologist or trichologist, can assist in identifying the underlying reason and formulating an individualized treatment regimen.

Chapter Three

Essential diet for hair development

Eating a balanced diet is essential for maintaining your hair's general health and stimulating hair growth. The following foods and vital nutrients can help with hair development:

PROTEIN: Since protein makes up the majority of hair, it's critical to consume enough of it in your diet. Lean meats like chicken, turkey, fish, eggs, dairy products, legumes, nuts, and seeds are all excellent sources of protein.

OMEGA-3 FATTY ACIDS: These fatty acids assist in nourishing and stimulating hair follicles. Omega-3-rich foods include walnuts, soybeans, chia seeds, flaxseeds, and fatty fish, including salmon, trout, and sardines.

ANTIOXIDANTS: Antioxidants assist in shielding hair follicles from the harm that free radicals can inflict. Consume a diet rich in fruits and vegetables, such as leafy greens, tomatoes, oranges, grapes, and berries.

VITAMINS: A number of vitamins are essential for healthy hair development, including:

- *Vitamin A:* aids in the production of sebum, which hydrates the scalp. Carrots, sweet potatoes, kale, spinach, and liver are some examples of sources.

- *Vitamin C:* promotes the synthesis of collagen, which fortifies hair fibers. Broccoli, bell peppers, strawberries, kiwis, and citrus fruits are good sources.

- *Vitamin E:* promotes better blood circulation to the scalp and functions as an antioxidant. Rich sources of vitamin E include avocado, nuts, seeds, and spinach.

- ***B-Vitamins (Biotin, B6, B12):*** Crucial for scalp health and hair growth. Incorporate foods such as dairy products, leafy greens, meat, poultry, fish, eggs, and whole grains.

MINERALS: A few minerals are essential for hair strength and growth.

IRON: aids in supplying hair follicles with oxygen. Red meat, chicken, fish, beans, lentils, spinach, and fortified cereals are good sources.

ZINC: promotes the development and restoration of hair. Zinc-rich foods include chickpeas, cattle, lamb, oysters, and pumpkin seeds.

SELENIUM: promotes the health of the scalp. Good sources include meat, fish, whole grains, dairy products, and brazil nuts.

COLLAGEN: This is a structural protein that supports hair development and structure. Collagen supplements, fish, chicken skin, bone broth, and other foods can increase the body's collagen levels.

HYDRATION: To keep your hair hydrated and your general health in check, you must drink enough water. Try to consume eight glasses of water or more each day.

It is important to note that maintaining a balanced diet that consists of a diverse range of foods that are high in nutrients is crucial for stimulating hair growth and maintaining your hair's health. In addition, ensuring optimal physical well-being through consistent physical activity, effective stress control, and appropriate hair care routines also plays a significant role in promoting healthy hair development. If you possess particular apprehensions regarding your hair or dietary habits, it is advisable to get guidance from a healthcare expert or a certified nutritionist.

Factors that contribute to hair growth

Numerous factors affect hair development, including genetics, hormones, the environment, and lifestyle. The following are some of the main elements that support hair growth:

GENETICS: Genetics largely influences hair growth patterns, including hair thickness, texture, and growth rate. Your genetic composition primarily determines your hair growth cycle and maximum hair length.

BLOOD CIRCULATION: Healthy blood flow to the scalp provides vital nutrients and oxygen to hair follicles, encouraging the creation of new hair. You can achieve improved scalp circulation through scalp massages, consistent exercise, and avoiding tight hairstyles that obstruct blood flow.

NUTRITION: The key to encouraging healthy hair

development is a well-balanced diet full of vital nutrients. An adequate intake of protein, vitamins (particularly B-vitamins, vitamin A, vitamin C, and vitamin E), minerals (such as iron, zinc, and selenium), and omega-3 fatty acids supports optimal hair development and follicle health.

SCALP HEALTH: The condition of your scalp directly impacts hair growth. An ideal environment for hair follicle growth is a clean, well-moisturized scalp free from ailments like dandruff, scalp psoriasis, or fungal infections.

HORMONES: Variations in hormone levels can have an impact on hair growth. Dihydrotestosterone (DHT), a derivative of testosterone, and other hormones can affect the activity of hair follicles, especially in cases of androgenetic alopecia (male and female pattern baldness). Hormonal changes during puberty, pregnancy, menopause, or thyroid diseases can also impact hair growth cycles.

STRESS LEVELS: Prolonged stress can cause excessive shedding or hair loss by interfering with the hair development cycle. Healthy hair development can be preserved by controlling stress using relaxation techniques, consistent exercise, getting enough sleep, and getting advice from friends or experts.

HAIR CARE PRACTICES: Using heat styling equipment excessively, getting chemical treatments too harshly, wearing tight hairstyles, and handling hair roughly can weaken hair follicles and damage the hair shaft, which can result in breakage and stunted growth. Adopting appropriate hair products, practicing gentle hair care, and avoiding over-manipulation can promote healthy hair development.

AGE: As people age, their hair growth tends to slow down, and their growth cycle may shorten. People may experience a decline in their hair growth rate and weaker hair as they age.

DRUGS AND MEDICAL CONDITIONS: Certain drugs, medical procedures like chemotherapy, and underlying medical conditions like autoimmune diseases, hormone imbalances, and nutritional deficiencies can impact hair growth. To address these concerns, it could be important to consult with a healthcare provider.

Hair infections and disorders

Hair disorders and infections can damage the scalp and hair follicles, causing a variety of symptoms and diseases. The following are some typical infections and hair disorders:

RINGWORM

A ring-shaped mark appears on the skin as a result of a fungal infection called ringworm. Ringworm can affect any part of the body, including the scalp.

Tinea capitis is the term for ringworm that affects the scalp. Anywhere on the scalp, ringworm can result in a red, scaly patch of baldness. These spots may seem brown or grayish on darker skin types. This may cause numerous distinct patches to appear all over the scalp. Children are more likely than adults to get ringworms on their scalps.

A person can contract the virus via another person, an animal, or a moist environment, such as a public pool. People should avoid sharing towels or other personal objects with someone who has ringworm in order to lower the risk of contracting the disease.

SEBORRHEIC DERMATITIS

This prevalent skin disorder is characterized by flaky, dehydrated skin. Seborrheic dermatitis may itch and produce redness. It can also result in darker skin tones with black patches and blotches.

A baby's scalp may develop cradle cap, which is a type of seborrheic dermatitis. In adults, the most typical cause of dandruff is seborrheic dermatitis.

SCALP PSORIASIS

An immune system malfunction causes long-term psoriasis, a skin disorder. Psoriasis on the scalp affects 45–56% of individuals with the condition, according to one study. Patches on white skin are often thick, red, and sometimes covered in silver scales. Hispanics are more likely to have silvery-white scales with salmon-colored psoriasis, whereas African Americans typically have violet-colored psoriasis with gray-colored scales.

FUNGAL INFECTIONS

Rarely, an environmental fungus may cause a fungal infection on the scalp. Mucormycosis, an uncommon infection brought on by fungi found in soil, is one example. Fungus can enter the body through breaks in the skin, such as cuts or skin conditions. Among the symptoms are:

- blisters or ulcers on the skin

- redness

- pain

- warmth around the infection

Fungal infection patches usually seem paler on darker skin types.

Individuals with compromised immune systems are more vulnerable to fungal infections. People who have cuts or damaged skin should cover and clean them to lower their risk of fungal infections. This is especially important when working in or near dirt.

FOLLICULITIS

Hair follicles are where body and scalp hair grow.

Bacteria that penetrate the skin through broken hair follicles can cause a condition known as folliculitis.

People may contract scalp folliculitis from:

- shaving or hair removal from the scalp

- frequently touching the scalp

- wearing tight hats or other headgear prolonged periods of hot, damp skin

When someone has follicullitis, a crimson ring surrounds every hair follicle. Rather than appearing red, darker skin types may have gray or brown pimples instead. This could itch or cause pain.

IMPETIGO

Impetigo is a common skin disease that often affects children. It is a bacterial infection that spreads easily. Although Staphylococcus germs are generally benign, they have the potential to spread infection if they get into injured skin.

The bacteria Streptococcus can also cause impetigo. This bacteria can spread from one person to another through sneezing, coughing, skin-to-skin contact, and item contact.

When the skin breaks, impetigo can affect any part of the body, but it typically affects the face, particularly the area around the mouth and nose. This also includes the scalp. Impetigo can also spread to other parts of the body from its original location.

Red lesions on the skin that rupture and leave a yellow-brown crust are the result of impetigo. In darker skin tones, the redness could be more difficult to perceive and appear more dark red, purple, brown, or gray. Large, fluid-filled blisters that burst open and leave discomfort can also result from it. These blisters and sores can hurt and frequently itch.

LICHEN PLANUS

Lichen planus, a skin ailment that results in glossy, reddish-purple plaques, affects white skin. On darker skin tones, it may appear more purple, brown, or black, and there is no noticeable scaling. On the scalp, lichen planus development is uncommon. However, when it does manifest on the scalp, it typically leads to:

- redness

- skin irritation

- losing hair in the affected area

- reddish-purple bumps

SCLERODERMA

Scleroderma is a disorder in which the body produces too much collagen. As a result, the skin becomes tighter and tougher than usual. Although the cause of this rare disease is unknown, there may be connections to the immune system. Usually, a line on the face or scalp indicates the disappearance of the tissue beneath the thicker skin.

TRICHOTILLOMANIA

The psychological condition known as trichotillomania is characterized by the need to pull out one's hair, which results in bald patches and substantial hair loss. People frequently use it as a stress or anxiety coping technique.

Chapter Four

Recommended alkaline meals for promoting hair growth

Some advocates say that consuming alkaline foods might enhance general well-being and potentially assist with specific conditions, such as promoting healthy hair. An alkaline diet aims to preserve the body's pH balance by consuming foods that are predominantly alkaline, such as fruits, vegetables, nuts, seeds, and legumes. Avoid or limit acidic items such as meat, dairy, processed meals, and caffeine.

Nevertheless, there is a lack of compelling scientific evidence establishing a direct correlation between alkaline diets and hair growth. A range of factors, including heredity, hormonal equilibrium, food consumption, and overall well-being, determine the health of one's hair.

The Top 12 Foods to Increase Hair Growth

1. Berries for collagen synthesis and antioxidants

Berries are rich in vitamins and other healthy components that may promote hair growth. Among these is vitamin C, which possesses potent antioxidant qualities. Antioxidants have the ability to shield hair follicles from the damaging effects of free radicals. Both the environment and the body naturally contain these chemicals. For example, one cup (144 grams) of strawberries has 85 milligrams, or up to 113% of your daily vitamin C requirements. Moreover, the body uses vitamin C to produce collagen, a protein that helps strengthen hair and prevent it from breaking and becoming brittle.

Moreover, vitamin C facilitates the body's absorption of iron from food. Low iron levels can lead to iron deficiency anemia, a condition associated with hair loss.

2. Eggs for protein and biotin

Two important nutrients for hair growth are protein and biotin, both of which are abundant in eggs. Protein makes up the majority of hair follicles, so eating enough of it promotes hair growth. Hair loss may result from a protein deficiency. Because keratin, a protein found in hair, depends on biotin for its formation, biotin supplements are frequently sold as hair development aids. For those who lack biotin, biotin can promote hair growth. However, if you eat a balanced diet, biotin deficits are rare. There isn't much data to support the idea that increasing biotin intake is beneficial for those with few or no health problems. Although it is unlikely that you will eat too much biotin, there is biotin above the daily recommended intake in many supplements for the growth of hair, skin, and nails. Zinc, selenium, and other elements that are good for hair health are also abundant in eggs. As a result, they are among the best nutrients for the healthiest possible hair.

3. Sweet potatoes to obtain beta-carotene

Beta-carotene can be found in sweet potatoes. The body converts this substance into vitamin A, which is associated with healthy hair.

About 114 grams, or a medium sweet potato, has enough beta-carotene to meet up to 160% of your daily requirements for vitamin A. Studies have indicated that vitamin A can impact sebum production, which contributes to the maintenance of healthy hair. A deficit in vitamin A may cause hair loss. However, excessive vitamin A consumption may also lead to hair loss.

Eat foods high in vitamin A, such as sweet potatoes, and try not to use too many supplements in order to meet your needs.

4. Spinach for iron, folate, vitamin C, and vitamin A

A nutritious green vegetable, spinach is full of iron, folate, and vitamins A and C, all of which are vital for good hair growth. Studies indicate that vitamin A plays an important role in hair growth.

However, using excessive amounts of vitamin A supplements might cause hair loss. Eating meals high in vitamin A should provide you with all the required amounts of this essential mineral.

Spinach makes up to 20% of your daily need for vitamin A in just one cup (30 grams). Furthermore, spinach is rich in iron, which is essential for healthy hair growth. Iron supports growth and repair as well as your metabolism by assisting red blood cells in transporting oxygen throughout your body. A shortage of iron may cause hair loss.

5. Fatty fish for protein and omega-3 fatty acids

Nutrients found in fatty fish, such as mackerel, herring, and salmon, may encourage hair development. They are rich in omega-3 fatty acids, which may promote the growth of hair. In a previous trial involving 120 female participants, a supplement containing antioxidants and omega-3 and omega-6 fatty acids reduced hair loss and enhanced hair density.

On the other hand, the literature on omega-3 fatty acids and hair development is very limited. It will need further research before medical professionals can prescribe anything. Aside from being an excellent source of protein, selenium, vitamin D3, and B vitamins, fatty fish may also aid in supporting strong, healthy hair. Hair loss and vitamin D3 insufficiency have been related in several studies. It's a good idea to consistently consume fatty fish and other sources of vitamin D in your diet, even though it's still uncertain if low vitamin D causes hair loss.

6. Seeds for zinc, selenium, and vitamin E

Seeds have few calories and are high in nutrients. Numerous nutrients also aid in the growth of hair. Selenium, zinc, and vitamin E are a few of these. An ounce (28 grams) of sunflower seeds contains a variety of B vitamins that are good for hair health, as well as about half of your daily vitamin E requirement.

Some seeds, like chia and flaxseeds, also contain omega-3 fatty acids.

There are 4.7 grams of omega-3 fatty acids in two tablespoons of ground flaxseed. The body doesn't absorb the form of omega-3 fatty acid in flaxseeds as well as it does in fatty fish. Still, they are a fantastic supplement to the diet. It is important to eat a variety of seed types to acquire the greatest range of nutrients.

7. Avocados for vitamin E and healthy fats

Avocados are a great source of healthy fats, as well as

tasty and nutritious.

They are also a good source of vitamin E, which may promote hair growth. About 200 grams, or one medium avocado, supply 28% of your daily need for vitamin E. Similar to vitamin C, vitamin E functions as an antioxidant to counteract free radicals and reduce oxidative damage. Some studies have identified reduced amounts of vitamin E in patients suffering from hair loss, although the evidence is inconsistent. In a previous study, taking a vitamin E supplement for eight months increased hair growth by 34.5% in participants who were experiencing hair loss. Additionally, vitamin E shields the scalp and other skin regions from oxidative stress and damage. Damaged scalp skin can lead to reduced hair follicle count and poor hair quality.

8. Nuts for zinc, vitamin B, vitamin E, and healthy fats

Nuts are delicious, handy, and packed with several nutrients that support healthy hair development. For instance, one ounce, or 28 grams, of almonds meets 48% of your daily requirement for vitamin E. They also supply zinc, important fatty acids, and a range of B vitamins. A deficiency in any of these nutrients could contribute to hair loss.

Beyond just promoting hair growth, nuts have also been connected to other health advantages, including lowered inflammation and a lower risk of heart disease.

9. Sweet peppers to boost vitamins A and C

Vitamin C from sweet peppers is high in antioxidants and may promote hair growth. A single yellow pepper can meet up to 456% of a woman's daily vitamin C requirements and 380% of a man's. Vitamin C increases the production of collagen, strengthening the hair strands. Additionally, it is a potent antioxidant that may shield hair strands from oxidative damage. Free radicals overwhelm the body's antioxidant defense mechanism, leading to oxidative stress. Studies have linked it to both hair graying and hair loss.

Sweet peppers are also a good source of vitamin A.

This vitamin influences the production of sebum, which keeps hair healthy and is crucial for hair development.

10. Oysters to get zinc

Oysters are one of the best zinc-rich foods to eat. A single medium oyster can provide up to 96% of a female's daily zinc requirements and 75% of a male's.

Zinc is one mineral that supports the hair growth and repair cycle.

Telogen effluvium, a frequent but reversible kind of hair loss brought on by a lack of nutrients, may be encouraged by a diet low in zinc. Zinc deficiency-induced hair loss may be counteracted by taking a zinc supplement. But an excess of zinc can be harmful. That is why eating foods like oysters may be preferable to taking supplements because they contain zinc in small but healthy levels.

11. Beans for zinc, protein, and other nutrients

Beans are an excellent plant-based source of protein that is necessary for hair growth.

Similar to oysters, beans are an excellent source of zinc, which supports the cycle of hair development and repair. A serving of 3.5 ounces (100 grams) of black beans can meet up to 14% of a woman's daily zinc requirements and 10% of a man's. They also supply iron, biotin, and folate, among many other minerals that are beneficial to hair health. In addition to all of these advantages, beans are cheap and incredibly flexible, making them a simple addition to any diet.

12. Soybeans to produce spermidine

Studies have linked compounds in soybeans to increased

hair growth. Soybeans contain large amounts of spermidine, one of these substances.

A trial involving 100 participants found that a nutritional supplement based on spermidine extended the anagen phase, during which hair is actively growing. A hair follicle will grow longer if it remains in the anagen phase long. Spermidine may encourage the growth of human hair, according to other studies. However, further research is required before medical professionals may prescribe spermidine intake because the relationship between spermidine and hair development is still relatively new.

Chapter Five

DIY processes for making hair growth shampoo

Green tea with honey recipe

Since dandruff can lead to hair loss, this green tea and honey mixture may promote hair growth. Honey also works wonders as a moisturizer for dry hair.

Ingredients:

2 tbsp. of honey

1 tsp. of olive oil

½ of cup green tea

¼ of cup castile soap

1 tsp. of lime juice or aloe vera

5–10 drops of peppermint and lavender essential oils

Instructions:

- Tea bags or green tea leaves can be brewed.

- Mix thoroughly after adding the green tea to the remaining ingredients.

A recipe using aloe vera

If your hair seems dry and brittle, try this aloe vera DIY shampoo recipe. Aloe vera reduces hair loss by balancing the pH level of the scalp, while almond oil relieves scalp irritation.

Ingredients:

½ cup castile soap

½ cup water

⅓ cup aloe vera

4 tbsp. almond oil

Instructions:

- Mix every component together.

Carrot with Maple Recipe

This homemade shampoo recipe with carrot and maple is another option for hair growth. This 2016 study found that while maple syrup has antibacterial qualities and helps prevent dandruff and nourish your hair, carrot oil naturally contains antifungal effects that promote hair growth.

Ingredients:

15 drops of carrot seed essential oil

15 drops of castor oil

3 tbsp. maple syrup

½ cup castile soap

Instructions:

- Blend every ingredient until it is smooth.

Almond with Aloe Vera Recipe

This shampoo might work best for you if your hair is dry and brittle. Aloe vera reduces hair loss by balancing the pH level of the scalp, while almond oil relieves scalp irritation.

Ingredients:

½ cup of liquid castile soap

½ cup of water

1/3 cup of aloe vera gel

4 tablespoons of almond oil

Instructions:

In a container, combine all the ingredients, then massage into wet hair for three minutes.

DIY processes for making hair growth cream

Shea Butter Hair Cream

Ingredients:

All-natural shea butter

An oil of your choice (e.g., almond oil, coconut oil)

Instructions:

- Gently melt the shea butter.

- Stir in the same quantity of your preferred oil after the shea butter has melted.

- Blend the mixture until smooth.

- After washing, use the cream as a leave-in treatment on the tips of your hair.

Shea butter with coconut oil recipe

Ingredients:

Pure shea butter

Coconut oil

Beeswax

Instructions:

- In a double boiler, first melt the beeswax, coconut oil, and shea butter.

- After they have melted, remove them from the fire and mix in the essential oil and apricot kernel oil.

- Transfer the blend into a glass jar or other container and let it cool. After it has cooled, use it as needed to preserve and treat your hair.

Chapter Six

Alkaline smoothie recipes that enhances hair growth

Strawberry with Spinach Smoothie

This energizing drink is one of the best alkaline morning smoothies. It gives you steady energy to keep you energized all day. Leafy greens (like spinach) that are dark and rich in nutrients are essential for blood pressure reduction, improved bone health, and easier digestion. On the other hand, strawberries have a high antioxidant content that can help prevent a number of diseases and conditions.

Ingredients

2 cups of spinach

½ cup strawberries

1 lime

1 banana

1 cup of coconut water

1 tbsp. hemp seeds

Preparation

Put all the ingredients in a blender and process them until they are smooth and creamy. You can use a frozen or fresh banana. Instead of putting the whole lime in the blender, squeeze out the juice. You can add stevia to the smoothie to enhance its sweetness.

Kale and Berry Smoothie

If you would like an alkaline smoothie that will provide you with energy throughout the rest of the day, you might consider making this delicious drink. The main ingredient in this dish, kale, is well known for having the highest nutritional content of any food on the planet. This vegetable is a great source of protective antioxidants. It can offer defense against cancer and heart problems. Strawberry and raspberry eating also has the ability to improve short-term memory and cognitive attention. Berries have the potential to improve brain function by changing the way neurons communicate with one another.

Ingredients

1 cup of kale

1 piece of banana

½ cup strawberries

1 cup of orange juice

¼ cup raspberries

Preparation

You can get the bananas, strawberries, and raspberries fresh or frozen. Pour the ingredients into a blender and add a few ice cubes to make it even more refreshing.

Avocado and Almond Milkshake

Having a smoothie or snack after working out is essential for refueling your body. With almond butter and almond milk, this alkaline smoothie packs a lot of protein. This macronutrient is essential for promoting muscle repair following exercise. Conversely, avocados contain a wealth of healthy fats that can rejuvenate your appearance and improve the absorption of any fat-soluble nutrients you eat.

Ingredients

1 avocado

1 tbsp. raw almond butter

1 cup of almond milk

1 banana

1 tbsp. chia seeds

Preparation

You can use coconut or hemp milk in its place if almond milk isn't your thing. Pick between a frozen banana and a peeled banana. Blend the ingredients until they reach a smooth consistency.

Cucumber and Kiwi Smoothie

Kiwi is popular because of its unique and enticing flavor. Kiwi is not only a delicious fruit, but it is also very nutrient-dense. This fruit protects the DNA in your cells from oxidative damage. It can also strengthen your immune system and successfully control your blood pressure. Cucumbers also help you stay hydrated, support cardiovascular health, and may even help you lose weight.

Ingredients

1 kiwi fruit

¼ cucumbers

½ bananas

1 handful of spinach

3-4 almonds

¼ cup coconut milk

Preparation

Combine all of these items in a blender. To further boost the cooling effects of this alkalizing smoothie, add a few ice cubes to the blender.

Watermelon and Cucumber smoothie

This watermelon smoothie is alkalizing, so get ready to feel rejuvenated. Watermelon and cucumbers are well-known for their hydrating and alkalizing qualities. This smoothie is ideal for an afternoon pick-me-up or breakfast.

Ingredients

2 cups of fresh watermelon chunks

1/2 cucumber

1/4 cup of fresh mint leaves

1 tablespoon of chia seeds

1 cup of coconut water

A drizzle of agave nectar (optional for added sweetness)

Preparation

Fill your blender with all the ingredients, then process

until smooth. Savor the alkaline watermelon smoothie!

Tricks for the best alkaline smoothies ever!

Let's speak about some expert advice to make sure you create the ideal alkaline combination before you turn on your blender.

1. Choose the freshest ingredients possible.

Avoid grabbing the wilted spinach located in the rear of the refrigerator. When making alkaline smoothies, freshness is essential! Select colorful, crunchy vegetables and luscious, ripe fruits. With fresher components, your food's flavor and nutrients will improve.

2. Harmonize alkalinity and flavor.

Alkalinity is important, no doubt, but flavor is equally important. In your blender, striking the correct balance is like producing a symphony of flavors. Start with greens that are alkaline, such as spinach or kale, and then sweeten with fruits. Do you need some zing? Squeezing some lime or lemon helps.

3. Select the appropriate blender.

Invest in one that can effortlessly handle even the most difficult fruits and greens. With a good blender, your smoothie will be silky smooth and free of chunks that are annoying.

4. Store all the ingredients for your alkaline smoothie properly.

Prepare the ingredients ahead of time! Prepare produce by washing, chopping, and freezing it in portion-sized bags. It guarantees that your smoothie is cold without requiring ice, saving you time. Store ingredients like leafy greens in sealed containers to preserve their crispness and freshness.

5. Alkali-based ice cubes can be made.

Use cucumber or lemon slices to flavor water and freeze it to create alkaline ice cubes. These cubes will keep your smoothie frozen while adding an extra dose of alkalinity.

6. Steer clear of typical alkaline smoothie errors.

Finally, avoid typical enticements. Don't use excessive amounts of sugars or acidic elements, such as citrus.

Chapter Seven

Top 10 Alkaline Hair Enhancing Recipes

A Quinoa Salad Dressed in Citrus Vinegar

Ingredients:

1 cup of cooked quinoa

Mixed greens (such as spinach, kale, and arugula)

1 orange, segmented

1/4 cup sliced almonds

1/4 cup diced red onion

Dressing: One tablespoon each of fresh lemon juice and honey, two teaspoons of olive oil, and salt and pepper to taste.

Instructions:

- Combine the cooked quinoa, diced red onion, sliced almonds, mixed greens, and orange segments in a large bowl.

- To create the dressing, whisk the olive oil, lemon juice, honey, salt, and pepper in a small bowl.

- Drizzle the salad dressing over it, then toss to coat. Serve and savor your revitalizing, high-alkaline meal.

Salmon Baked with Roasted Veggies

Ingredients:

2 salmon fillets

Diced root vegetables (carrots, sweet potatoes, and beets)

1 tablespoon olive oil.

Chopped fresh herbs (such as thyme or rosemary)

To taste, add salt and pepper.

Instructions:

- Preheat the oven to 375°F (190°C).

- Place the salmon fillets on a baking sheet lined with parchment paper.

- In a separate bowl, combine diced root vegetables, olive oil, chopped herbs, salt, and pepper.

- Arrange the seasoned veggies around the salmon fillets on the baking sheet.

- Bake for 15 to 20 minutes, or until the veggies are soft and the salmon is cooked through, in the preheated oven.

- For an alkaline-rich and delectable meal, serve the baked fish with roasted veggies.

Alkaline Fruit Mix

Ingredients:

Walnuts

Almonds

Pumpkin seeds

Unsweetened dried cranberries

Goji berries

Instructions:

- In a bowl, combine equal amounts of goji berries, pumpkin seeds, walnuts, almonds, and dried cranberries.

- Divide the fruit mix into tiny snack packs for easy on-the-go munching.

- Enjoy your high-nutrient, alkaline snack whenever you're hungry.

Alkaline Green Drink

Ingredients:

A handful of spinach

1/2 cucumber

1/2 avocado

1 banana

1 cup of almond milk

1 tablespoon of chia seeds

Instructions:

- Blend all of the ingredients until smooth.

- Enjoy your nutrient-rich, alkaline drink after pouring it into a glass.

Walnut with pumpkin seeds smoothie

Ingredients:

1 tbsp. pumpkin seeds

1 tbsp. walnuts

1 small banana

2 tbsp. oats (cooked and chilled)

½ cup almond milk or coconut water

½ cup avocado

Instructions:

- Blend all the ingredients together.

- Serve and enjoy your creamy smoothie.

Blackberries and avocado mix

Ingredients:

¾ cup mangoes

¾ cup blackberries

¾ cup avocado

½ tsp. lemon juice

¾ cup water

Instructions:

- Mix each ingredient in a blender until smooth.

- Savor your mix.

Fruity Mix

Ingredients:

¾ cup spinach

¾ cup orange juice

¾ cup strawberries

¾ cup banana

¾ cup almond milk

1 tbsp. chia seeds

Instructions:

- In a blender, purée the fruits with almond milk.

- Pulse once or twice after adding chia seeds, and then serve.

Cantaloupe smoothie with carrots

Ingredients:

½ cup, chopped carrot

½ cup, chopped, cantaloupe

¼ teaspoon Himalayan pink salt

Mint leaves

½ of one large grapefruit pulp

Instructions:

- Blend the grapefruit, carrot, and cantaloupe pulp with Himalayan pink salt.

- Pour some into a glass.

- Leafy mint is a nice garnish.

- Savor your refreshing smoothie

Kiwi-Orange Smoothie

Ingredients:

1 large orange

2 kiwi, chopped with the peel

½ cup watermelon

A pinch of Himalayan pink salt

2 tablespoons of lime juice

Instructions:

- Blend together orange, kiwi, watermelon, lime

juice, and Himalayan pink salt.

- Pour the mixture into a mason jar to take with you wherever you go.

Smoothie with berries, dates, and walnuts

Ingredients:

½ cup of blueberries

¼ cup of raspberries, chopped

½ cup of blackberries

2, chopped dates

1 tablespoon of crushed walnut

Instructions:

- Blend together the dates, blueberries, blackberries, and raspberries.

- Pour the contents into a glass.

- Toss in the chopped walnuts just before serving.

In addition to tantalizing your taste buds, these delicious recipes nourish your hair from the inside out, giving you the glowing locks of your dreams. Accept the benefits of an alkaline diet, and watch as your hair gleams with life and energy.

ACKNOWLEDGEMENTS

All glory belongs to God. I'd also want to thank my wonderful family, partner, fans, readers, friends, and customers for their constant support and words of encouragement.